D0027714

Chapter 1

(Re)-introduction

Welcome to the second installment of "Unreported Truths."

This section will focus on the evidence lockdowns do - or don't - reduce the spread of the coronavirus. I also will examine the failure of the models that forecast virus patients would overrun hospitals. Their erroneous predictions play a crucial role in explaining whether lockdowns are effective.

But first, some background.

I've had a strange few weeks. Maybe you have too.

On Wednesday, June 3, I finished editing Part 1 of "Unreported Truths," about coronavirus death counts. I decided to publish the booklet through Amazon's self-publishing platform, Kindle Direct Publishing. I'd written twice for an Amazon program called "Kindle Singles," where the company publishes pieces from professional writers. So, although I knew Unreported Truths might anger some people in the media, I figured Amazon would be fine with it.

After all, Amazon sells "Mein Kampf" and "The Anarchist's Cookbook" and "Bestiality and Zoophilia: Sexual Relations with Animals." As it should. Amazon should not judge the books on its digital shelves, except in very rare cases where they offer specific advice on criminal behavior. Amazon seems to agree it should err on the side of making books available. In a statement in April, a company spokesman wrote that "As a bookseller, we believe that providing access to the written word is important, [including] books that some may find objectionable."

https://www.propublica.org/article/the-hate-store-amazons-self-publishing-arm-is-a-haven-for-white-supremacists

I also knew nothing in Part 1 could be considered a conspiracy theory. Nearly all the data in it comes from published scientific papers and official government sources. So when I uploaded Part 1 to the Kindle Direct site on Wednesday night, I figured I'd see it for sale on Amazon the next morning.

Wrong. When I checked KDP in the morning I found the book, which had been listed as being "In Review," had been returned to "Draft" status. Then Amazon emailed me:

> Your book does not comply with our guidelines. As a result we are not offering your book for sale... **Please consider removing references to COVID-19 for this book.** [Emphasis added.]

Obviously, I would have a tough time removing references to COVID-19 in a book about COVID-19.

I was shocked. Besides the company's supposed commitment to free speech, Amazon had benefitted hugely from the coronavirus lockdowns, which had forced many competitors to close. Its stock was at an all-time high, giving it an astronomical value, more than $1 trillion. (It has risen even higher since.) Under the circumstances, I thought Amazon had a special obligation to let people offer criticisms of the lockdowns. Apparently not.

I considered making the book available through my Website, but Amazon has a huge share of both the e-and physical book markets. And Amazon can sell, print, and deliver books faster than anyone else. Traditional publishers told me they would need up to a month to get the pamphlet out. Amazon could make copies available in days. I *needed* access to Amazon's audience.

I knew trying to force Amazon's hand would probably fail. The company is notoriously unresponsive to criticism. Still, I figured making noise couldn't hurt. What could Amazon do, ban the book? It already had. I went to Twitter, where my contrarian stance on lockdowns had gained me more than 100,000 followers. (Okay, that number was not even 0.2 percent as many as Kim Kardashian had, but I hoped it still might be enough to help a little.)

My heartfelt if less than eloquent plea: "Oh fuck me. I can't believe it. They censored it – " above a screenshot of the Amazon rejection email.

A number of conservative writers quickly spoke up against Amazon's censorship. So did a few on the left, notably Glenn Greenwald of The Intercept. Greenwald wrote that although he disliked my views on Covid, "book banning by corporate tech giants is a far worse danger than whatever threats [Unreported Truths] supposedly presents."

But reporters at traditional media outlets – including friends at The New York Times, *where I had worked for a decade* – mostly stayed quiet. Their silence baffled and disheartened me. Some said explicitly Amazon's audience simply shouldn't have the chance to see the booklet – a view that cuts against every idea of intellectual freedom.

By 1 p.m., I was worried. I figured if I couldn't get Amazon to pay attention by the end of the day, I might have to distribute the book myself.

Then Elon Musk stepped up.

Again.

Musk and I have still never met or even had a phone call. Maybe we never will. But if we do, I will buy him a beer (not that he needs me to buy him a beer). In the unlikely event you haven't heard of Musk, he's the chief executive of Tesla and SpaceX and has tens of millions of followers on Twitter. He is unafraid to speak his mind, and he views the lockdowns as a catastrophic mistake. He'd retweeted me before, and we had been in touch over text sporadically since early May.

I told Musk what had happened. Just before 2 p.m., he spoke up, as only he can – posting below my original tweet, "This is insane." He followed up with a second tweet, "Time to break up Amazon. Monopolies are wrong."

Musk's comments put a spotlight on Amazon's censorship. The Wall Street Journal, CNBC, and even the Washington Post – which Bezos owns – wrote articles. And someone at Amazon got the message. At 2:59 p.m., 65 minutes after Musk's tweet, I received an email from "Kindle Direct Publishing – Executive Customer Relations" telling me Amazon would publish Part 1.

Maybe Amazon would have backed down anyway. I don't know. But Musk's throwdown surely sped the process. (Amazon told reporters it had banned "Unreported Truths" in error, but it never said so to me. And it continues to ban COVID-19 books. As far as I can tell, the only error it made was censoring someone with a big enough megaphone to fight back.)

The kicker to the story came that night, after I appeared on Fox News and One America News to talk about the censorship and the booklet. I checked my Amazon sales page and found that over the course of an hour the book had sold almost *10,000* digital copies – more than two every second. By midnight it had sold 26,000. It briefly hit #1 in the Kindle Store. It has now sold more than 130,000 paper and ebook copies worldwide.

In other words, Amazon's censorship almost certainly gave "Unreported Truths" a boost. But though I was lucky, censorship by big technology companies is a growing problem. Most people who get banned aren't going to have Elon Musk to speak for them.

Meanwhile, the United States was on fire.

Through early June, the death of George Floyd sparked the most serious race-related demonstrations since the Rodney King riots of 1992. Media outlets pivoted to full-time coverage of the protests. By day, protesters filled Minneapolis, New York and other cities. By night, rioters looted stores.

The anger was real and understandable. But I assumed – wrongly, as it turned out – that the protest coverage meant the media's coronavirus hysteria was over.

The reason was simple.

The epidemic was fading across most of the world. European countries had reopened without problems. In the United States, southern states had begun to reopen more than a month earlier – Georgia on April 24, Texas not long after – without much trouble. Even in the Northeast, the hardest-hit region, states were edging towards partial reopenings. Hospitals were closing COVID-specific units and instead getting back into the business of elective surgeries and other ordinary health care.

Newspapers and cable networks were reduced to hyping case counts in countries like Peru, or writing speculative articles about potential post-infection syndromes. The most troubling example came in May, as reporters focused on a disease in children that looked very much like Kawasaki disease, which can lead to serious heart problems in kids. The New York Times led the way, writing more than a dozen articles in May. Its headlines quickly moved from claiming the illness might be "related to" coronavirus to calling it a "baffling virus syndrome."

https://www.nytimes.com/2020/05/13/health/coronavirus-children-kawasaki-pmis.html

https://www.nytimes.com/2020/05/05/nyregion/kawasaki-disease-coronavirus.html

Never mind that the syndrome appeared very rare and showed up in some kids who had not even had coronavirus infections. Never mind that the official British Kawasaki disease society repeatedly discounted the link. On May 15, the society wrote, "With continuing sensationalist press pieces causing deep worry for families, we wanted to share another paper... Children are unlikely to be seriously affected by Covid-19 infection." https://www.societi.org.uk/kawasaki-disease-covid-19/pims-ts/

And never mind that even in serious cases of the inflammatory syndrome, most children recovered quickly after steroids or other immuno-suppressive therapy. As a Texas pediatric infectious disease expert told a television station in Austin, "'In general, most of these kids do fine.'" Which didn't stop the station from headlining its June 3 story, "Deadly illness in children linked to COVID-19 confirmed in Austin hospital."

https://www.kvue.com/article/news/health/coronavirus/multisystem-inflammatory-syndrome-dell-childrens-austin-coronavirus/269-ef12525f-213c-437a-ad9a-094f422c2f99

For months, I had referred to articles hyping the dangers of Covid as "panic porn" (and people writing them as members of "Team Apocalypse"). The Kawasaki articles were worse, frightening parents based on the thinnest possible science. I called them "kiddie panic porn," an ugly name for an ugly media game.

Yet the stories also hinted at the media's desperation to find bad news as the epidemic waned. Thus when the Floyd protests exploded I imagined the media would move away from Covid doomsaying.

I was wrong.

Since mid-June the number of positive tests for Sars-COV-2 has surged across the Sunbelt. In Florida, for example, daily positive tests rose 15-fold over a three-week period – from 617 on June 3 to more than 9,500 on June 27. Since then they have risen still further.

Many factors, both real and testing-related, are driving the rise. Restaurants are open. Voluntary social distancing has relaxed. Hot summer weather has driven people inside and increased reliance on air conditioning, which may help spread the virus. The Floyd protests and migration from Mexico may also have played a role, though those factors are more speculative.

Meanwhile, testing has skyrocketed. Some employers are requiring tests before employees can return to work. Hospitals are testing everyone who comes in for elective surgeries. The result has been a huge surge in positive tests, which the media insists on calling "cases." But using the word "case" implies someone has a clinically significant illness – that they are sick enough to need hospitalization or at least medical attention. In fact, many people infected with the coronavirus do not even know they have it, especially if they are under 50 and in decent health. They most often have either no symptoms at all or a low fever or cough, symptoms indistinguishable from a bad cold or mild flu.

Thus the increase in positive tests has far outstripped any increase in hospitalizations, intensive care admissions, ventilator use, or deaths. Every death – from Covid or any cause – is a tragedy. But for now coronavirus deaths remain significantly lower than they were in the Northeast in March and April. And we have every reason to think that they will stay that way. The vast majority of the new cases are in people under 60, who are at much lower risk. And since mid- to late July, hospitalizations have declined sharply in Arizona, Texas, and Florida – the states that led the increase.

Unfortunately, the media remains as devoted to hysteria today as in March. And the Sunbelt spike has given journalists new fuel for the panic. We are hurtling towards a fall without normal schools, while lockdowns are starting again. On July 13, California governor Gavin Newsom once again closed bars, gyms, indoor restaurant service, houses of worship, and other services.

California has about 40 million people. Since the epidemic began almost five months ago, the state has had about 9,000 deaths from the virus, *none* in anyone under 18. That's correct: Not one person under the age of 18 has died in the largest American state from Sars-Cov-2. Yet California's economy and society remain crippled.

Two big media-fed misrepresentations – I won't call them lies – work in concert to drive our policies.

First, the media has hidden the reality that anyone who is not extremely elderly or sick has a miniscule risk of dying from the coronavirus. In Part 1, Inon offered the real numbers and risks, based on the best government data. And since Part 1 was published, even more studies have emerged. A new Swedish government report puts the risk of death from Sars-Cov-2 at 1 in 10,000 for everyone under 50 – including those who have chronic conditions.

And in a talk on July 14, Dr. Robert Redfield, the director of the Centers for Disease Control, put the risk of deaths in children under 18 at 1 in 1 million. https://www.buckinstitute.org/covid-webinar-series-transcript-robert-redfield-md/ Major media outlets simply ignore this data.

But the media's *other* distortions are arguably even more important. Beginning in March, news outlets demanded lockdowns and lauded the public health experts who pressed for them. The few governors who resisted faced enormous pressure. A typical New York Times article from early April was headlined, "Holdout States Resist Calls for Stay-at-Home Orders: 'What Are You Waiting For?'" (https://www.nytimes.com/2020/04/03/us/coronavirus-states-without-stay-home.html)

The scrutiny extended to entire nations, such as Sweden. (https://www.cnn.com/2020/04/28/europe/sweden-coronavirus-lockdown-strategy-intl/index.html)

What went all-but-unnoticed in the push for lockdowns was the fact that major public health organizations had for decades *rejected* them as a potential solution to epidemics. In just the last three years, the Centers for Disease Control and the World Health Organization have published new epidemic planning manuals with specific recommendations about what to do if respiratory viruses hit.

The CDC published its guide in 2017, while the WHO's is even more recent and detailed. (https://www.cdc.gov/mmwr/volumes/66/rr/rr6601a1.htm)

(https://apps.who.int/iris/bitstream/handle/10665/329438/978
9241516839-eng.pdf?ua=1) Dozens of scientists and physicians
worked on the WHO's guidelines, reviewing laboratory studies,
clinical trials, and real-world evidence. The manual runs 91
pages, plus a 125-page annex with the details of the "literature
reviews" used to make the recommendations.
(https://apps.who.int/iris/bitstream/handle/10665/329439/WH
O-WHE-IHM-GIP-2019.1-eng.pdf?ua=1)

The CDC and WHO manuals don't mention Sars-Cov-2, of
course. It didn't exist when they were written. They focus on
influenza epidemics. But the flu and the coronavirus are both
respiratory viruses, and they are similarly infectious. So the
recommendations in them should apply broadly to Sars-Cov-2.
(The coronavirus is somewhat more lethal than the average flu
strain but *less* lethal than some strains the WHO report
anticipates.)

What's so striking about the manuals is how *little* they find
effective. Even when they make recommendations – for
handwashing, say, or "respiratory etiquette" (a fancy way to say
"coughing into your elbow") – they acknowledge little evidence
supports them. The endorsements are often made on the basis
that interventions are "acceptable," "feasible," and have few
"resource implications."

In other words, people can be taught to cough into their elbows
and will do so without complaining. So let them try. It can't
hurt. This theory extends at least partway to masks. (I'll come
back to masks in a future booklet. Despite the lack of evidence
for them, they have become uniquely important symbolically as
a way for the media and politicians to shame people who
challenge the official narrative that Sars-Cov-2 is an
extraordinarily dangerous disease.)

What about lockdowns?

Both the CDC and WHO found little reason to recommend them. The 2017 CDC planner did not even mention widespread workplace closings. It discussed school closings only as a temporary measure during "severe, very severe, or extreme pandemics."

Meanwhile, the WHO report also highlighted concerns about the costs of lockdowns, noting, in language only a bureaucrat could love, that "workplace measures and closures could affect the economy and productivity of a society." It "conditionally" recommended minor measures such as "staggering shifts, and loosening policies for sick leave." It added that "workplace closure should be a last step only considered in extraordinarily severe epidemics and pandemics" – such as Spanish flu-style outbreaks that might kill "millions" of people. In other words, not the coronavirus.

Yet when Sars-Cov-2 arrived in force in Europe and the United States in March, public health authorities ignored their own cautious advice. They played a frenzied tune that the media amplified loudly enough to drown out any competing voices.

In a matter of days, dozens of countries that supposedly valued individual rights and democratic freedoms had jumped into an experiment in state control unlike any since at least World War 2.

And the lockdowns began.

Chapter 2:

Lockdowns, then

In theory, lockdowns can slow or even stop epidemics.

In theory.

Understanding what lockdowns actually *are* is crucial. Media outlets often use the terms lockdown, quarantine, and social distancing interchangeably. But to public health experts they are very different. Scientists use the term "quarantine" to describe confining people exposed to someone else with an infectious disease. Those quarantined people aren't even necessarily sick, but they might be. The person who actually has the disease is properly said to be not quarantined but "isolated."

A lockdown is a broader response, perhaps more accurately described as a "mass quarantine," covering a community, state, or even country. It can include canceling public gatherings like sporting events and closing schools or workplaces. In a worst-case scenario, it can even extend to ordering everyone to stay at home. It may be enforced by a national border closure or "cordon sanitaire," a police or military-enforced boundary around a region to prevent anyone from entering or exiting.

In contrast, the phrase "social distancing" generally refers to *voluntary* measures that governments encourage but don't require, like working from home. But – confusingly – journalists and even public health experts sometimes use "social distancing" as an umbrella term to include mandatory measures.

Isolation. Home quarantine. Mass quarantine. Cordon sanitaire. "Safer-at-home." "Stay-at-home." Workplace closures. Staggered shifts. Telecommuting. Essential workers. School dismissals. School closures. Lockdowns. Mitigation. Suppression. The menu of terms is in its own way telling, evidence of the choices governments must make as epidemics spread.

Of all those choices, mass lockdowns are the most powerful and disruptive.

They are also the most seductive for policymakers, at least at first, because they seem so certain to work. Like influenza, Sars-Cov-2 is a respiratory virus transmitted through relatively large droplets of virus-riddled saliva and phlegm as well as smaller particles of raw virus – so-called droplet and airborne transmission. The droplets typically stay afloat only a few feet before falling to the ground, though the airborne particles can remain aloft for longer. Flu and coronavirus can also be passed through "fomites," viral particles people pick up by touching contaminated surfaces.

Keep people far enough away from each other, and all those "vectors" of transmission should be reduced, if not eliminated entirely.

In theory.

Scientists use one simple but crucial number to determine how fast an epidemic is spreading. They call it the reproduction number, or R. It measures the number of people a newly sick person infects in turn. If R is 1, each infected person infects on average *one* other person before losing the ability to pass the virus along. If R is greater than 1, an epidemic is growing. If it is less than 1, the epidemic is dying out.

A famous shampoo ad called "And They Told Two Friends" illustrates the principle: 1 becomes 2 becomes 4 becomes 8 becomes 16 becomes 32... until everyone in the world is using Faberge shampoo. https://retroist.com/and-they-told-two-friends-how-faberge-organics-shampoo-explained-virality/

Small differences in R can make huge differences to how quickly an epidemic spreads. That is especially true in the case of respiratory viruses, which have short transmission cycles. (In other words, they make people sick quickly, but those people are infectious for only a few days.)

For example, if each person infects two more over the course of a five-day transmission cycle, a single infection will spread to more than 100 people in a month. But if each person infects three others, then a single infection will become more than 700 in a month.

But R can change dramatically and quickly, and it does not depend solely on the virus itself. Transmissibility varies over time and from place to place. Many factors can change it, both natural and human-controlled. For example, influenza viruses typically don't do well in hot weather or strong sunlight, which is why flu season typically runs from October to March. Population density is another obvious factor. The higher it is, the better chance the virus has to jump from person to person. Viruses will mutate on their own, too. In general, mutations that make the virus more transmissible but *less* dangerous to its hosts will help the virus survive better over time.

The goal of a lockdown is to reduce R – to slow the transmission rate. Ideally, a lockdown would cut R below 1, so the epidemic shrinks instead of growing. But even a lockdown that merely *slows* the growth of an epidemic – reducing R from 3 to 2, for example – can help, by reducing strain on hospitals.

When policymakers use the phrase "flatten the curve," that's what they really mean. People will still be infected, and some will still die. But the disease will spread over a longer period. So hospitals will function more normally, including continuing to treat sick people who *don't* have the virus.

Imagine a theoretically complete lockdown. Everyone must stay at home for 90 days, no matter what. Get sick? Too bad, you stay home. Need to work? Too bad, you stay home. Drones deliver food and medicine. Anyone caught outside is immediately returned home (or, in the truly dystopian version of this story, shot). Thus the virus can only spread within people living in the same house, or maybe apartment buildings with shared ventilation systems. Everyone who gets it will either recover or die by the time the lockdown ends.

Eureka, no more virus.

Obviously, even this vastly oversimplified version of the "perfect" lockdown has holes. What if the virus survives in the same animal hosts where it hid before it jumped to people? What if some people are still sick at the end? What if the virus somehow remains dormant in some people until the lockdown is over? A little-known incident at a British Antarctic base more than 50 years ago suggests just how hard suppressing respiratory viruses can be.

In 1969, six researchers at the base developed moderate to severe cold symptoms. What made the incident so fascinating was that they got sick in the middle of the Antarctic winter, after they had been isolated from all human contact for *17 weeks straight*.
(https://www.ncbi.nlm.nih.gov/pmc/articles/PMC2130424/?page=10)

"The symptoms occurring in six of 12 men were totally unexpected," scientists wrote in a 1973 paper in what at the time was called *The Journal of Hygiene* (today it is known as *Epidemiology and Infection,* a name change that neatly captures the importance of cleanliness in slowing disease). If viruses can survive winter in Antarctica, what chance does even the strictest lockdown have?

In reality, we'll never know. Because in reality, the technology to enable such a stringent lockdown doesn't exist. Drones and robots can't farm or deliver food without human help. Unless the military plans to deliver rations to everyone, private food chains must keep running. Doctors and nurses have to work. So do power plant and communications workers, prison guards and police officers. And of course scientists to monitor the virus and work on treatments.

In a modern society, the list of essential workers rises fast. Outside of dystopian science-fiction thrillers, lockdowns can *never* be complete, or even close.

In democratic nations like the United States, the obstacles to a hard lockdown are even higher. Efforts to force people to stay inside are legally problematic. Governors must instead rely on fear and public pressure. But people will resist – to protect their rights, out of boredom, or because they need to work.

Thus American lockdowns focus less on police enforcement and more on closing businesses, schools, parks, entertainment venues like movie theaters, and government offices. When there's nowhere to go except grocery stores and Wal-Mart, many people will decide leaving their houses is not worth the trouble.

How many people will stay in and how many go out? The answer depends in part on how strictly governments enforce their rules. The lockdown China imposed on Hubei province in January was far stricter than even the strictest American lockdowns, with European countries in the middle. French authorities imposed almost a million fines, averaging more than $150, in the first month of that country's lockdown. (https://www.thelocal.fr/20200423/french-police-hand-out-over-900000-in-lockdown-fines-including-to-holiday-home-owners)

But under any circumstances, lockdowns reduce contact between strangers, possibly by as much as 75 percent.

So in March, as the Sars-Cov-2 epidemic jumped to Europe and the United States, epidemiologists and public health experts told governments to lock down – fast and hard. Not just mass gatherings, but schools, offices, malls, even parks and beaches. To do anything less would be to sentence millions of people to death, the experts said.

Most infamously, the Imperial College London report of March 16 – written by researchers who were working with the World Health Organization – predicted more than 2 million American coronavirus deaths without immediate action. It called for a policy of what Professor Neil Ferguson, the report's lead author, termed "suppression":

> [S]uppression will minimally require a combination of social distancing of the entire population, home isolation of cases and household quarantine of their family members. This may need to be supplemented by school and university closures...

(https://www.imperial.ac.uk/media/imperial-college/medicine/sph/ide/gida-fellowships/Imperial-College-COVID19-NPI-modelling-16-03-2020.pdf)

(Of course, Professor Ferguson exempted himself from his mandate. Two weeks after the report came out, as the entire United Kingdom had locked down, and *while Ferguson himself was still supposed to be self-isolating after contracting the coronavirus,* he had an affair with a married woman who traveled across London to meet him.)

The stunning impact of the Imperial College report made Ferguson arguably the most important public health expert in the world. Yet he was neither physician nor virologist. His PhD was in theoretical physics, arguments about the structure of the universe that are something close to pure math.

But he and the other Imperial College researchers appeared to believe a handful of relatively simple equations would predict the coronavirus epidemic. To be correct, the modelers would have to understand not only how the virus spread but the complex behavioral changes lockdowns would inevitably produce. Yet the models are hardly based on *any* real data about either spread *or* lockdowns.

At their core, these models are simply software programs designed to simulate reality, based on the assumptions that the person who creates them inputs into them. They are as realistic as a game of SimCity, though less colorful.

Nonetheless, Ferguson's model produced highly precise answers. Lockdowns could reduce coronavirus deaths 95 percent or more if they continued until a vaccine was developed. Ferguson and his team even offered different death projections based on the severity of the lockdowns and benchmarks used to lift and reinstate them.

These details gave the Imperial College model an undeserved sense of certainty and reliability. In this sense, they were like other mathematical simulations of real-world events – like the ones that assumed housing prices could never collapse across the entire United States at once and thus helped cause banks in 2006 and 2007 to miss the real-estate and financial crisis they were fueling.

But for all the complexity of his equations, Ferguson really offered nothing more than an updated version of the original frightened rationale for the quarantines European city-states had imposed during the Black Death seven centuries earlier: *Keep strangers away and we'll be safe.*

The idea of using widespread lockdowns to slow epidemics took off in 2006, as The New York Times reported in April:

> Fourteen years ago, two federal government doctors, Richard Hatchett and Carter Mecher, met with a colleague at a burger joint in suburban Washington for a final review of a proposal they knew would be treated like a piñata: telling Americans to stay home from work and school the next time the country was hit by a deadly pandemic.
>
> When they presented their plan not long after, it was met with skepticism and a degree of ridicule by senior officials...

(To be clear, the Times was *lauding* Drs. Hatchett and Mecher and their work justifying lockdowns. https://www.nytimes.com/2020/04/22/us/politics/social-distancing-coronavirus.html)

After a flu scare in 2005, then-President George W. Bush asked scientists for research on slowing epidemics. Dr. Mecher, an internist at the Department of Veterans Affairs, connected with Robert Glass, a computer scientist at Sandia National Laboratories. For a science project, Glass's 14-year-old daughter had created a model of the way social distancing might slow the spread of the flu. Glass built on it to create a simulation "proving" lockdowns could reduce an influenza epidemic in a hypothetical town of 10,000 people by 90 percent. "Dr. Mecher received the results at his office in Washington and was amazed," the Times wrote.

Robert and Laura Glass ultimately became the first two authors on a paper published in *Emerging Infectious Diseases,* a Centers for Disease Control journal, about the simulation. Inevitably, it contained a shout-out to Neil Ferguson. And sure enough, it showed the "mitigation strategies" worked.

In the retelling of this heroic lockdowns-for-all story by the Times, the conclusions of the paper took the CDC by storm. "In February 2007, the C.D.C. made their approach — bureaucratically called Non-Pharmaceutical Interventions, or NPIs — official U.S. policy."

The Albuquerque Journal told a similar tale about its hometown heroine in a May article:

> [Laura Glass's] work motivated research that resulted in the social distancing and self-isolation policies now being

> used to curtail the spread of COVID-19.
>
> "The inspiration, the sparks came from my daughter," said Robert J. Glass, a retired Sandia National Laboratories senior scientist. Glass was among those who built on Laura Glass's project to develop the vital strategies that are employed today.

(https://www.abqjournal.com/1450579/social-distancing-born-in-abq-teens-science-project.html)

The reality was different.

The 2007 CDC paper ran 108 pages and included descriptions of many possible ways to reduce transmission, from "voluntary isolation of ill adults" to "reducing density in public transit." (https://stacks.cdc.gov/view/cdc/11425)

Crucially, it also contained a "Pandemic Severity Index" that included five categories. On the low end, Category 1 represented a normal seasonal flu season, which still might kill up to 90,000 Americans. On the high end, a Category 5 pandemic, like the Spanish flu, would kill at least 1.8 million Americans.

Based on the CDC's scale, Sars-Cov-2 almost certainly should be classified as Category 2 epidemic, meaning it will cause between 90,000 and 450,000 deaths. For Category 2 or 3 epidemics, the CDC merely said governments should *consider* school closures of less than four weeks, along with moderate efforts to reduce contacts among adults, such as encouraging telecommuting.

The prospect of closing all retail stores or offices *is not even mentioned in the paper* – not even during a Category 5 epidemic killing millions of people. (The CDC's 2017 guidance, which superseded the 2007 paper, is less detailed but follows similar broad outlines. Crucially, the updated guidance lacked the "Pandemic Severity Index," ultimately giving public health officials and politicians more leeway to impose extraordinary measures.)

Yet the Times glossed over these distinctions in its article. It wrote instead "the (Bush) administration ultimately sided with the proponents of social distancing and shutdowns" and claimed the coronavirus response came directly from the original CDC report. "Then the coronavirus came, and the plan was put to work across the country for the first time."

Even as the CDC was putting its 2007 plan together, many scientists and physicians with expertise in treating pandemics worried about the weakness of real-world evidence for lockdowns and other interventions – and a potential overreliance on computer modeling.

Among the most vocal critics of lockdowns was Dr. Donald Henderson. Henderson, a recipient of the Presidential Medal of Freedom, led the successful effort to eradicate smallpox. In December 2006, Henderson and three others wrote an 11-page paper called "Disease Mitigation Measures in the Control of Pandemic Influenza." After outlining potential lockdown measures, they wrote, "We must ask whether any or all of the proposed measures are epidemiologically sound... [and] consider possible secondary social and economic impacts."

(https://www.liebertpub.com/doi/10.1089/bsp.2006.4.366?url_ver=Z39.88-

2003&rfr_id=ori%3Arid%3Acrossref.org&rfr_dat=cr_pub++0pub
med&)

Efforts in past epidemics to slow – much less stop – the spread
of the flu had largely failed, the authors wrote. They attacked
quarantines, travel bans, and school closings of more than two
weeks as likely counterproductive. They did not even mention
full lockdowns, presumably because they viewed those as so
unlikely. Near the end of the paper, they made a heartfelt plea:

> Experience has shown that
> communities faced with
> epidemics or other adverse
> events respond best and with
> the least anxiety **when the
> normal social functioning of
> the community is least
> disrupted.** [Emphasis added.]

Henderson and his co-authors were not alone in their concerns.

In 2006, the Institute of Medicine – a federally chartered non-
partisan group that offers advice on tough health questions –
held a conference to discuss flu outbreaks. Ultimately, the
institute produced a 47-page report on "modeling community
containment for pandemic influenza."

(https://www.nap.edu/catalog/11800/modeling-community-
containment-for-pandemic-influenza-a-letter-report)

The report repeatedly discussed the limitations of the research
on how epidemics spread. "A major limitation of the models is
the uncertainty in many of the assumptions," the report's
authors wrote. "There is little evidence to support many of the
key parameters."

At best, "models should be viewed as aids to decision-making, rather than substitutes for decision-making," the report warned. Unfortunately, "there is a real risk that in the midst of a crisis, there will be pressure for government to employ public health interventions, even in the absence of proven benefits."

These fears have proven prescient. And public health experts themselves were not only not immune to the panic, in many cases they seemed to lead it. Among Donald Henderson's co-authors on the 2006 paper was Dr. Thomas Inglesby, an infectious disease specialist and director of the Center for Health Security at Johns Hopkins University.

Inglesby didn't seem to change his views on lockdowns much over the next 14 years. On January 23, 2020, even as the coronavirus broke out in Hubei province, he tweeted his fear that "large scale quarantine for nCoV [the novel coronavirus] will be ineffective and could have big negative consequences." (https://twitter.com/t_inglesby/status/1220335490374742017)

Then, suddenly, he made a 180-degree turn. By April 6, he told Scientific American that the newly imposed lockdowns in the United States should not be lifted without "declines in new cases, widespread testing... and the use of nonmedical masks by the public." (https://www.scientificamerican.com/article/when-can-we-lift-the-coronavirus-pandemic-restrictions-not-before-taking-these-steps/)

I emailed and tweeted at Inglesby to ask if he saw any contradiction between the 2006 paper and his current stance, and if so how he explained the change in his views.

He did not respond.

But Inglesby was not alone in his sudden change of heart. As *The New York Times* reported in an April article about the British response to the coronavirus, top British scientists – including Neil Ferguson and the government's chief scientific advisor, Sir Patrick Vallance – had believed the United Kingdom would not need a lockdown. "Then, confronted with new numbers that projected hospitals would be overwhelmed with patients and that the death toll would skyrocket, they pivoted to a suppression strategy." (https://www.nytimes.com/2020/04/23/world/europe/uk-coronavirus-sage-secret.html)

The early March reports of overwhelmed hospitals in northern Italy – and Italy's aggressive response – no doubt played a role. On March 9, Italy began a hard national lockdown, becoming the first country to close its entire territory. All non-essential travel was banned. Stores and government offices were shut. Police began checking more than 100,000 people a day, and thousands were fined. (https://www.theguardian.com/world/2020/mar/18/italy-charges-more-than-40000-people-violating-lockdown-coronavirus)

Lost in the panic was the fact that Italy has had several recent severe flu epidemics. In both the 2014-15 and 2016-17 flu seasons, so-called influenza-like-illnesses killed more than 40,000 Italians – the equivalent of nearly a quarter-million Americans. Northern Italy appears to be particularly susceptible to respiratory viruses because it has a very elderly population and high levels of air pollution. (https://www.sciencedirect.com/science/article/pii/S026974912032060 1?via%3Dihub)

As the epidemic accelerated across Europe, Spain became the next major country to announce a lockdown, on Friday March 13. At that point, Imperial College still had not yet publicly released its paper projecting millions of deaths. But it had already been shown to politicians and policymakers in the United States and Europe.

"An Imperial College coronavirus model has had a profound impact on public policy since its results were shared with British and American officials **last week** [emphasis added]," the Financial Times reported on March 19. Ferguson had presented an estimate of 500,000 British deaths to a semi-secret British government scientific committee as early as February 27.

(https://www.ft.com/content/16764a22-69ca-11ea-a3c9-1fe6fedcca75)

(https://www.theguardian.com/world/2020/may/29/sage-minutes-reveal-how-uk-advisers-reacted-to-coronavirus-crisis)

The apparent success of the Chinese lockdown in quelling the epidemic in Hubei province may also have encouraged governments to consider stronger steps, although serious questions have been raised about the accuracy of the hospitalization and fatality data from China.

Journalists and historians will be sorting through the March panic for years. Only when governments fully declassify meeting notes and emails will we gain a more complete picture of what happened.

But the most likely explanation is the simplest. Faced with a risk of hundreds of thousands or millions of deaths, the public health experts who for decades had counseled patience and caution flinched. They found they could not live with acknowledging how little control they or any of us had over the spread of an easily transmissible respiratory virus. They had to do *something* – even if they had been warning for decades that what they were about to do would not work and might have terrible secondary consequences.

So lockdowns spread country to country and state to state. Even at the time, it was not clear whether the measures were intended to "flatten the curve" – to slow the spread temporarily and give hospitals a chance to get ready for a spike in cases – or to suppress the epidemic forever. No matter. The media cheered. Politicians vowed not to impose lockdowns, then changed their minds in days.

No one reversed course faster or harder than New York governor Andrew Cuomo. On Thursday, March 19, he promised that he would not impose a quarantine on his state:

> New York, and New York City in particular, will not be quarantined or force people to stay "locked up" in their homes or shelter in place. "None of that is going to happen," he said.

(https://www.nbcnews.com/health/health-news/live-blog/2020-03-19-coronavirus-news-n1163556/ncrd1163936)

The next day, Cuomo imposed a lockdown. (https://www.nydailynews.com/coronavirus/ny-coronavirus-cuomo-20200320-qrsrtcp3grfyvj5llf47cj6xoa-story.html) As he put it: "When I talk about the most drastic action we can take, this is the most drastic action we can take."

He was right.

Which didn't mean it would work.

Chapter 3:

Lockdowns, now

Too late.

We'd locked down too late.

As stores and offices and schools shut, as the United States braced for a surge, the fear in the media and from politicians was palpable; *the lockdowns hadn't come in time.* In New York City, the number of newly hospitalized patients with coronavirus more than tripled from 185 on March 15 to 665 on March 20. Everyone expected many more hospitalizations and deaths were coming, in New York and everywhere else. The only question was how many.

Why?

Because hospitalizations lag infections, and deaths lag hospitalizations.

Following infection with Sars-Cov-2, the average time to develop symptoms like fever or cough is five days. (https://www.ncbi.nlm.nih.gov/pmc/articles/PMC7081172/) Most people then recover relatively fast. But some get sicker. Within five to eight days, they need hospitalization. For an unlucky few, intensive care follows a day or two after, then intubation and death. In all, in the tiny fraction of cases when the novel coronavirus kills, death comes at roughly 18 days after symptoms begin and 23 days after infection. (https://www.thelancet.com/journals/laninf/article/PIIS1473-3099(20)30243-7/fulltext)

As the Atlanta Journal-Constitution explains, "epidemiologists agree that today's counts are a snapshot of what the virus did roughly two weeks ago. It can take a week or more for a person to become infected, show symptoms, get tested, and have their results reported."

(https://www.ajc.com/news/coronavirus-georgia-covid-dashboard/jvoLBozRtBSVSNQDDAuZxH/)

In other words, the people hospitalized in New York on March 20 had likely gotten sick before March 10. And they were the tip of the iceberg. The city hadn't closed schools until Monday, March 16. Offices and stores remained open during that week. But people who were infected on the 20th wouldn't show up at hospitals until the end of the month.

No one knew just how quickly infections had increased between March 10th and 20th, but the potential numbers were terrifying. Hospitalizations had risen 3.6-fold in five days. If they increased again at that rate over the next 10, the city would have almost 9,000 patients *a day* by March 30 before the lockdowns finally kicked in.

Thus Cuomo projected that coronavirus patients would soon overrun every medical center in New York. On Tuesday, March 24, he projected New York would need 140,000 hospital beds and 40,000 ventilators for them within two to three weeks – an unfathomable catastrophe.
(https://www.cnbc.com/2020/03/24/gov-cuomo-says-new-york-needs-ventilators-now-help-from-gm-ford-does-us-no-good.html).

These doomsday projections proved far off. But Cuomo wasn't making them on his own. The hospital center Weill Cornell Medicine, the consulting firm McKinsey & Company, and the

CDC were all advising him. And on March 26, the Institute for Health Metrics and Evaluation at the University of Washington released its own forecasts for all 50 states.

The IHME works closely with the Gates Foundation, which gave it $279 million in a 10-year-grant in 2017. Its mission statement says it "provides rigorous measurement and analysis of the world's most prevalent and costly health problems." Its model purported to forecast deaths, hospitalizations, and ventilator needs for every state and many countries.

IHME's forecasts predicted a terrifying future, with a sharp and unstoppable rise in cases. Within three weeks, the United States would need nearly 250,000 hospital beds for coronavirus patients, as well as more than 30,000 intensive care beds – far more than were available in many states.

Crucially, IHME released its model *after* most states had begun lockdowns, and the model assumed the shutdowns would continue until the epidemic was over. In fact, IHME assumed that even states which had not yet locked down would do so:

> [The forecasts are] predicated on the enactment of social distancing measures in all states that have not done so already within the next week and maintenance of these measures throughout the epidemic.

(http://www.healthdata.org/research-article/forecasting-covid-19-impact-hospital-bed-days-icu-days-ventilator-days-and-deaths)

Along with the rapid peak, the model assumed a quick plunge in hospitalizations after lockdowns took hold. By early May, hospitalizations nationally would fall under 100,000, and by late May below 30,000, it said.

(http://www.healthdata.org/sites/default/files/files/research_a rticles/2020/COVID-forecasting-03252020_4.pdf)

This forecast only made sense if *lockdowns worked to reduce transmission, quickly and certainly.* Like the Imperial College model, the IHME model assumed the epidemic would spread uncontrolled before hard lockdowns but rapidly shrink thereafter, as R – the transmission rate – fell below 1.

Overnight, the IHME model became the crucial forecasting tool for state and federal governments. On April 8, the Washington Post called it "America's Most Influential Coronavirus Model." (Any criticism came mostly from epidemiologists who believed its forecasts were too rosy.)

(https://www.washingtonpost.com/health/2020/04/06/americ as-most-influential-coronavirus-model-just-revised-its-estimates-downward-not-every-model-agrees/)

In the 10 days after the institute released the model, it repeatedly revised upwards its forecasts for hospitalizations and ventilator use. For example, on April 5, the revised IHME model projected that New York would need 69,000 hospital beds and almost 10,000 ventilators *that day.*

What no one in the media or at the Institute for Health Metrics and Evaluation seemed to care about – or even notice – was that the model had failed completely. It was failing not just to predict the future but accurately measure of what was happening *in real time.*

On April 5, New York actually had about 16,500 people in hospitals – fewer than one-quarter the number **the model**

claimed were hospitalized that day. Of those, about 4,000 patients, not 10,000, were on ventilators. (https://www.nbcnews.com/health/health-news/why-some-doctors-are-moving-away-ventilators-virus-patients-n1179986)

Why did the IHME model fail just days after it was released? Why did it and the other models so badly overestimate the number of patients who would be hospitalized with the coronavirus?

The institute and its director, Dr. Christopher Murray, did not return emails for comment.

But the simplest answer for the model's crucial initial failure is that growth in hospitalizations in New York slowed much faster than it forecast. After their 3.6-fold rise between March 15 and March 20, new admissions doubled again by March 25, to 1,323. Then their exponential growth abruptly ended.

Over the next two weeks, they stayed in the range of 1,300 to 1,700 a day, before beginning a rapid decline. (Overall hospitalizations actually peaked earlier and declined faster, as patients began to be discharged fairly quickly.)

In most other states, hospitalizations in late March never really accelerated. The model proved just as inaccurate everywhere else, though off a lower base.

An aside: no one can blame the failure of the models on lack of compliance with the lockdowns. All over the world, most people accepted the measures as unfortunate but necessary. Businesses, offices, and schools closed. Air travel nearly vanished. Even as the lockdowns stretched deep into April, most Americans and Europeans stayed home without much complaint.

A combination of fear, public pressure, and a genuine desire to support frontline health-care workers seems to have driven obedience. Heavy media and corporate propaganda helped. Endless television ads aimed to convince people to "come together by staying apart." (By mid-April, an advertising copywriter named Samantha Geloso had created a hilarious spoof, but that didn't stop the ads. https://adage.com/creativity/work/montage-takes-piss-out-pandemic-montages/2250301)

By mid-April, some Americans – mostly conservatives – had begun to demand an end to the lockdowns. But their protests made little difference. Media outlets like CNN and the Times, which fully supported the lockdowns, treated the protests as fringe events. They never gained enough momentum to matter. The governors who locked down their states the hardest saw the *biggest* jumps in their approval ratings.

Data from Apple on mobility shows how effective the lockdowns were. Across the United States, driving dropped 25 percent in the week before March 20, then fell another 50 percent before bottoming out on Sunday, April 12. Mass transit use bottomed the same day, down 80 percent from normal levels. (https://www.apple.com/covid19/mobility) Overall, American mobility dropped almost two-thirds from early March to mid-April before slowly recovering.

That figure was less than lockdown champions such as Italy – where the drop was more than 80 percent and lasted even longer – or the United Kingdom. But it was comparable to countries like Germany and higher than many people might have predicted before the lockdowns began.

Further, the national data don't catch the impact of the lockdowns in hard-hit areas. In New York City, driving bottomed out at 30 percent of normal, mass transit use at barely 10 percent. Even those figures underestimate the way the city *felt*. Hundreds of thousands of people fled New York in March and April. Aside from police officers, medical staff, and other essential workers, almost no one went outside. The empty streets and shuttered stores were eerie, as I saw for myself on repeated trips.

No, the failure or success of lockdowns can't be blamed on lack of compliance.

What, then? The IHME model and its cousins badly overestimated hospitalizations. But their failures didn't end with that error. They were wrong *both on the way up and the way down*. The models predicted a short peak and rapid decline, but hospitals emptied slowly.

And although the models overestimated hospitalizations, they *underestimated* the number and timing of deaths. In its various revisions, IHME predicted between 60,000 and 90,000 American deaths by August, with deaths falling sharply after a mid-April peak. The United States currently has about 150,000 reported deaths, and deaths both in the United States and elsewhere dropped only slowly.

In Britain, Ferguson made a similar mistake when he reduced his estimate of deaths from 500,000 to 25,000 on March 25. Britain has now had 46,000 deaths.

The simulations designed by the world's top epidemiologists failed in every way.

Why?

The most likely answer has everything to do with lockdowns. *The failure of the models cannot be separated from the failure of lockdowns.* Neil Ferguson and the epidemiologists designing the models believed that lockdowns worked, that they were the only way to make the epidemic manageable.

But they misunderstood the fact that lockdowns failed utterly to protect the people most at risk.

The worst coronavirus outbreaks have followed the same pattern everywhere – whether Wuhan in January, northern Italy in early March, or New York and London a few days later. In a densely populated area, Sars-Cov-2 spreads quietly but quickly for days or weeks – a Chinese researcher estimated that the R might have been close to 3.9 in Wuhan in January, a rate that if unchecked means 1 infection would become more than 3,000 in a month. (https://docs.google.com/presentation/d/1-rvZs0zsXF_0Tw8TNsBxKH4V1LQQXq7Az9kDfCgZDfE/edit#slide=id.p32)

The illness then jumps into public view as conventional and social media fill with doomsday predictions. And as a lockdown is considered, even if it is initially rejected, the panic rises still further. Although people may begin to travel less and voluntarily socially distance during this period, emergency room visits and 911 calls soar, driven both by fear and real viral spread.

In New York, emergency room visits for respiratory and flu-like symptoms rose from about 1,700 a day at the beginning of March to more than 4,000 by the middle of the month. Some people already had coronavirus or the flu. Others were simply afraid. For them, emergency rooms were an ideal ground to pick up or trade the virus. They also increase the risk of passing the virus to the physicians and medical staff who treat them – who in turn can spread it to patients who are already hospitalized.

This pattern rapidly became clear to front-line doctors. As early as March 21, a group of physicians in northern Italy warned in a New England Journal of Medicine article:

We are learning that hospitals might be the main Covid-19 carriers, as they are rapidly populated by infected patients, facilitating transmission to uninfected patients. Patients are transported by our regional system, which also contributes to spreading the disease as its ambulances and personnel rapidly become vectors...

[Sars-Cov-2] is not particularly lethal, but it is very contagious. The more medicalized and centralized the society, the more widespread the virus.

(https://catalyst.nejm.org/doi/full/10.1056/CAT.20.0080?fbclid=IwAR0wa6jzq-t_YYlZlYQtWiVmphT8pjyGBCndLhJGSN34dBaeZJoGP0sfneo)

In other words, panic itself drives vulnerable people to hospitals and thus increases transmission among them. And nothing causes panic to spike faster than the serious consideration of lockdowns.

At the same time, lockdowns force people to stay inside. (Obviously. That's the *point* of lockdowns.)

Unfortunately, coronavirus spreads most efficiently inside, especially in households living in poorly ventilated apartments or small houses, their windows closed against winter cold or summer heat. On March 30, Dr. Mike Ryan, the Irish surgeon who leads the World Health Organization's COVID containment and treatment program, warned at a WHO press conference:

> At the moment, in most parts of the world, due to lockdown, most of the transmission that's actually happening in many countries now is happening in the household at family level. In some senses, transmission has been taken off the streets and pushed back into family units.

(https://www.youtube.com/watch?v=2v3vlw14NbM&feature=youtu.be&t=2996, at approximately 50:00.)

[Ryan's solution to this problem was to propose forcibly isolating infected patients and quarantining their family members, but that's a story for another day, and a later section of Unreported Truths.]

All over the world, researchers and government agencies have reached the same conclusion. On April 7, Chinese researchers published a paper that looked at 318 outbreaks with 1,245 Sars-Cov-2 infections. They found that 80 percent took place in homes or apartments. Another 34 percent occurred on public transportation (some outbreaks occurred in more than one place, or could not be placed at a single venue). All other venues, including stores and restaurants, accounted for less than 20 percent of infections combined.

"Sharing indoor space is a major SARS-CoV-2 infection risk," the researchers wrote.

(https://www.medrxiv.org/content/10.1101/2020.04.04.20053058v1)

Similarly, in examining a week of cases from June 28 through July 4, the Health Ministry of Quebec reported fewer than 15 percent could be traced to workplaces, stores, or bars and restaurants. 35 percent were intra-familial. Another 25 percent were of health care workers, patients, or prison inmates, and a similar number could not be traced. Particularly striking about the Quebec figures is that they occurred after the province's lockdown had ended.

(https://www.cbc.ca/news/canada/montreal/covid-19-quebec-why-are-cases-increasing-1.5658082)

In other words, in the short run, increasing the amount of time family members spend with each other may drive up transmission.

Even worse, the people most vulnerable to that intra-familial transmission of coronavirus – the extremely elderly and people with severe health problems – rarely work and are the *least* likely to spend time outside. They are naturally somewhat protected, until lockdowns confine them with family members who have been infected elsewhere and bring the virus home.

Worst of all, broad lockdowns do not appear to make much difference to the spread of the virus in nursing homes. Long-term care facilities are uniquely vulnerable to the coronavirus because their patients are both medically fragile and live close together. Fewer than 0.5 percent of Americans live in nursing homes – fewer than 1 in 200 people. But in both the United States and Europe, nursing home residents have accounted for 40 to 50 percent of all Covid deaths, well over 100,000 in all. (https://www.theguardian.com/world/2020/may/16/across-the-world-figures-reveal-horrific-covid-19-toll-of-care-home-deaths)

Even during lockdowns, nursing homes and other "congregate care" facilities cannot close. How to protect them, then? Measures such as frequently testing staff members and patients, ensuring the homes have adequate cleaning equipment, and quickly hospitalizing infected residents may help contain outbreaks.

But the effort required to promote and manage lockdowns can distract governments from the crisis in nursing homes. In northern Italy, as a strict lockdowns dragged on, "nursing homes were in many ways left to fend for themselves," an Associated Press article reported on April 26. (https://www.whsv.com/content/news/Perfect-storm-Lombardys-virus-disaster-is-lesson-for-world-569961341.html) The panic that lockdowns foment may even play a role in causing staff to flee and leaving residents without care, as happened in Spain. (https://www.npr.org/sections/coronavirus-live-updates/2020/03/24/820711855/spanish-military-finds-dead-bodies-and-seniors-completely-abandoned-in-care-home)

The fact that lockdowns do little to help nursing homes may be one reason that deaths go on so long after they begin – contrary to the forecasts from IHME and others. The United Kingdom, which has had more deaths per-capita than any other big country, imposed a lockdown nearly as strict as Italy's on March 23. Deaths peaked April 10 at about 1100 a day, but remained around 630 a day almost four weeks later. And more than 16,000 of the deaths occurred in nursing homes.

Six months into the epidemic, the data are clear: the overall number of people infected with Sars-Cov-2 is less relevant to the number of people who die than *which people are infected*.

Only when nursing home and hospital outbreaks burn out do deaths decrease.

An April 15 paper from the Robert Koch Institute, Germany's equivalent of the Centers for Disease Control, offers a slightly different perspective on the issue.

In the paper, researchers there tracked the number of infections in Germany for more than two months. They found that the spread of the virus peaked at the beginning of March. At that point each newly person infected 3 others – an R of 3, showing just how contagious Sars-Cov-2 can naturally be. Over the next three weeks the transmission rate fell to around 1.

(https://www.rki.de/DE/Content/Infekt/EpidBull/Archiv/2020/Ausgaben/17_20_SARS-CoV2_vorab.pdf?__blob=publicationFile)

Yet Germany imposed a hard lockdown *late* – on March 23, two weeks after Italy's.

What happened? Southern Germany is not even 200 miles from the northern Italian border. Reports about the burgeoning outbreak in Italy apparently prompted Germans to take their own voluntary social distancing measures and reduce the spread of the virus – *before* the damaging panic that comes with the consideration and imposition of a lockdown.

The lockdown itself reduced the transmission marginally more, to 0.9. But it did little to protect vulnerable populations, the report warned. "After March 18 the virus spreads more to older people and we are also increasingly seeing outbreaks in nursing homes and hospitals."

Still, Germany made containing outbreaks in nursing homes a priority. And it wound up with a fraction of the nursing home deaths – or overall deaths – in Britain, Italy, or Spain.

(https://www.theguardian.com/world/2020/jun/28/covid-19-risk-of-death-in-uk-care-homes-13-times-higher-than-in-germany)

Yet more evidence that lockdowns were ineffective came after American states and European countries lifted them. Denmark was the first European country to end its lockdowns, reopening schools in April and stores by early May. More than a month later, on June 10, the Danish national health authority reported that "there is no sign yet of noticeable changes." Switzerland and other European countries noted similar trends.

(https://www.reuters.com/article/us-health-coronavirus-denmark/denmark-sees-no-rise-in-covid-19-cases-after-further-easing-of-lockdown-idUSKBN23H1DU)

In the United States, southern states began lifting lockdowns as early as April 24, led by Georgia. The decision led to predictable media hysteria. The Atlantic magazine infamously called the decision "Georgia's Experiment In Human Sacrifice."

Yet the United States saw no spike in coronavirus cases in May or early June. On May 20, Marko Kolanovic, a senior strategist at J.P. Morgan (like Neil Ferguson, a physicist by training), analyzed reopening and transmission data. He concluded that the virus had actually spread more slowly in the United States after lockdowns ended.

Then, in June, cases began to rise in a broad stretch of states from California to Florida. Hospitalizations followed. In Arizona, the first state to see a major spike, hospitalizations more than tripled from roughly 1,000 on June 1 to 3,500 on July 13. In Texas, the spike began later but was even sharper, from 2,000 on June 11 to almost 11,000 on July 22. Florida saw a similar trend, with hospitalizations rising from roughly 2,000 to almost 9,000.

Deaths also surged in all three states, though with a predictable lag. (Death reporting is tricky not just because the criteria for counting deaths as Covid-related are extremely loose but because some deaths are reported almost immediately while others are not counted for weeks or even months.) By any count, though, hospitalizations and especially deaths have occurred at a far lower level than the Northeast in March.

Several different and plausible explanations for the Sunbelt spike have been offered – including the heavy use of air conditioning, young people deciding not to protect themselves because they now know they are at low risk, and possibly even some importation of cases from Mexico. That confused reality has not stopped media outlets from insisting that the end of lockdowns must have been responsible for the rise in infections – even though the rise began between five and eight weeks after the lockdowns ended.

Even more importantly, the media has largely failed to report that the *Sunbelt spike in hospitalizations is over.* Arizona, Florida, and Texas have all seen big drops in hospitalizations in late July. The drop is most stunning in Arizona, where cases peaked first. Between July 13 and August 3, hospitalizations fell to just over 2,000 – a drop of almost 50 percent. In Texas, hospitalized Covid patients fell from their July 22 peak to under 9,000 by August 3, a drop of almost 20 percent. In all three states, hospitals were stressed, but none faced overrun and the overall quality of care either Covid or other patients received appeared unaffected.

Further, in all three states, the drop in hospitalizations came *despite the fact the states did not reimpose widespread lockdowns,* though they did take minor steps to slow the spread of the virus and reduce the strain on hospitals. Arizona closed gyms and bars, for example, while Florida closed bars and Texas postponed elective surgeries. (Neither Arizona nor Florida mandated masks, either, although Texas required them in most counties.)

About 180 years ago, a British epidemiologist and statistician named William Farr examined data from smallpox and other epidemics and concluded that in viral epidemics, deaths tend *to both rise and fall* in a roughly symmetrical pattern that looks like a bell curve – a long tail followed by a quick rise followed by a rounded peak, with a sharp drop and a long tail on the other side.

What's so striking about Farr's observation is that the type of virus and its lethality and transmissibility don't seem to matter as much as our (voluntary) human response to the virus – and the gradual growth in the number of people who have been infected by and recovered from the virus and can no longer pass it on. Further, Farr noted that epidemics generally strike the most vulnerable first and hardest: "The most mortal die out." As a result, early estimates of mortality may be hugely overstated.

(https://www.sciencedirect.com/science/article/pii/S2468042718300101)

(https://www.cebm.net/covid-19/covid-19-william-farrs-way-out-of-the-pandemic/#:~:text=Farr%20showed%20that%20epidemics%20rise,pattern%20on%20the%20downward%20slope.)

The shape of the hospitalization curves in Arizona couldn't fit Farr's law better – a bell curve with a rounded peak and a sharp drop. Lockdown or not, a simple theory did a far better job of predicting the course of the epidemic there than powerful computer simulations.

Any worldwide review of lockdowns must touch on three other countries: Sweden, New Zealand, and Japan.

Sweden has attracted a huge amount of attention as the only major Western European country to refuse to lockdown. At first glance, Sweden appears to provide evidence for both pro- and anti-lockdown views. Per-capita death coronavirus rates there are lower than Britain or Italy, though higher than Germany or the Nordic countries.

In fact, though, Sweden's high death rates were driven almost entirely by the fact that the country didn't just fail to protect nursing homes but in some cases actually discouraged physicians from offering care to the extremely elderly. In a June article headline, "Coronavirus Is Taking a High Toll on Sweden's Elderly. Families Blame the Government," *The Wall Street Journal* detailed disturbing cases in which older patients had been refused hospitalizations. (https://www.wsj.com/articles/coronavirus-is-taking-a-high-toll-on-swedens-elderly-families-blame-the-government-11592479430)

As a result, Sweden's coronavirus deaths skew extremely elderly. Almost two-thirds of deaths occurred in people 80 or over, and almost 90 percent in people 70 or over. The Swedish government has acknowledged that its failure to protect nursing homes was a huge and preventable error.

Overall, the course of the epidemic in Sweden has essentially tracked that of countries like Italy and Spain – a big early spike, followed by a slow decline. The trend suggests lockdowns are irrelevant, and that protecting nursing homes makes far more difference.

On the other hand, the most impressive country-level evidence in favor of lockdowns comes from New Zealand, which locked down very hard and very early, and now appears to have largely eliminated the coronavirus on its territory. But – like Newfoundland, a Canadian province that took similar steps – New Zealand is an exceptional case, a lightly populated and isolated island that plays a minor role in global commerce and can easily shut its borders.

Those states may be the *only* ones with a realistic chance of using lockdowns to control the coronavirus, as long as they are willing to enforce long-term border quarantines and aggressively track any positive case; whether the dangers of the virus justify such steps is a question more political than scientific. And even in those areas, any relaxation of the rules may lead to a quick spike in cases, as Hawaii – which until recently appeared to have controlled the virus effectively – is now learning.

If New Zealand offers the strongest case for lockdowns, Japan offers the opposite. Japan should have been ground zero for the epidemic. It has one of the world's oldest populations, one of its largest cities, heavy reliance on mass transit, and close air links to China. Its poor performance quarantining the ill-fated *Diamond Princess* cruise ship in February suggested its authorities lacked basic infection control awareness. "Health officials and even some medical professionals worked on board without full protective gear," the Times reported on Feb. 22. (https://www.nytimes.com/2020/02/22/world/asia/coronavirus -japan-cruise-ship.html)

And Japan never imposed a full national lockdown, instead in April imposing only a partial "state of emergency" that lasted only a few weeks and consisted of largely voluntary restrictions. As Bloomberg News wrote in May:

> No restrictions were placed on residents' movements, and businesses from restaurants to hairdressers stayed open. No high-tech apps that tracked people's movements were deployed. The country doesn't have a center for disease control. And even as nations were exhorted to "test, test, test," Japan has tested just 0.2% of its population -- one of the lowest rates among developed countries.

Yet Japan has had an almost bizarrely easy time with Sars-Cov-2. It has reported about 250 cases per million people, even fewer than New Zealand, and 8 deaths per million – about 1 percent of Britain's rate.

Why? No one really knows. Many Japanese wear masks in public, especially if they have fever or cough, although masking is far from universal. Authorities also discouraged people from gathering in crowds, in closed spaces like bars, and talking closely – the "three Cs" strategy.

(https://www.sciencemag.org/news/2020/05/japan-ends-its-covid-19-state-emergency?utm_campaign=news_daily_2020-05-26&et_rid=687438071&et_cid=3340566)

If those explanations seem unsatisfying, it's because they are. But we can be sure lockdowns are *not* the reason for Japan's success. Yet American public health experts have for the most part simply *ignored* Japan and simply continued to snipe at Sweden, rather than doing the hard work of grappling with their policy choices and apparent successes.

One last point: scientific journals have recently published several papers purporting to show that lockdowns saved hundreds of thousands or even millions of lives. Not to put too fine a point on it, these papers are junk – mathematical models created in some cases by the very same epidemiologists whose forecasts four months ago proved entirely wrong. And these models are even more useless, because they aren't even trying to predict the future but instead describing an alternative past that didn't take place and thus cannot be proven true or false.

For example, in June, Imperial College researchers (yes, again) put out a paper claiming that lockdowns might have saved *millions* of lives in Europe. Beyond the fact that the researchers used an estimate for the virus's risk of death far higher than the current best estimates, they looked at 10 European countries. They found that lockdowns, however and whenever they were exposed, had worked in all 10.

(https://www.nature.com/articles/s41586-020-2405-7)

But they included Sweden as a lockdown country.

Which unintentionally made the point exactly the opposite of the one they intended. After all, if Sweden had the same results as everywhere else, how can anyone think lockdowns made a difference?

Considered as whole, the evidence – at best – suggests hard lockdowns *may* eventually slow the general spread of the coronavirus. After all, following months of lockdowns, the epidemic in Italy, Spain, and New York did burn out.

Even that case is not proven, as Sweden shows. With or without lockdowns, some hard-hit countries and regions may eventually reach "herd immunity." Essentially, herd immunity occurs when so many people have already been infected and recovered and developed antibodies that the virus can no longer move freely through the population.

But the debate over what percentage of the population must be infected before herd immunity is reached is both highly technical and subject to many of the modeling uncertainties that have proven so damaging already. So it's best left for later.

What lockdown proponents seem to forget is a general gradual slowdown makes little difference, especially for a virus whose risks are as skewed to the elderly and sick as Sars-Cov-2. What matters is breaking spikes that can cause hospital overrun, while protecting the vulnerable. General lockdowns do neither. And because of the fear they provoke and the leadership attention they require to promote and implement, they are a distraction from focusing on those in need of protection at the worst possible time.

Even the WHO seems to have recognized the futility of lockdowns. In a recent interview with the British newspaper The Telegraph, Dr. Maria Van Kerkhove, a leader of the organization's coronavirus response team, discouraged countries from reimposing lockdowns. They are a "blunt, sheer force instrument" with severe social and economic consequences, she said.

(https://www.telegraph.co.uk/global-health/science-and-disease/exclusive-top-disease-detective-warns-against-return-national/)

Some European leaders have publicly admitted lockdowns were a mistake. In July, Jean Castex, the French prime minister, said the country would never again "impose a lockdown like the one did last March, because we've learned... that the economic and human consequences from a total lockdown are disastrous."

(https://www.france24.com/en/20200708-france-rules-out-total-lockdown-in-case-of-covid-19-surge)

Yes, the economic and human consequences. I thought I'd write a lot about those in this section, but I haven't bothered, because they are so self-evident. More than 50 million Americans have filed for unemployment; the United States economy shrank by 1/3 in the second quarter on an annualized basis, the sharpest drop ever recorded.

The damage goes far beyond bank accounts. Since March, drug overdose deaths have spiked from New Jersey to British Columbia; murders have soared in many big American cities. (We don't know exactly how much, because although we obsessively count coronavirus deaths in real-time, we pay far less attention to other causes of death.) Millions of "elective" surgeries have been postponed worldwide, leading to untold misery for patients suffering from chronic pain, failing joints, and other ailments, and even death in the cases of people needing heart surgery or cancer care.

(https://www.dailymail.co.uk/news/article-8396253/UK-patients-face-TWO-YEAR-wait-elective-surgery-NHS-backlog-set-hit-650-000.html)

(https://nowtoronto.com/news/april-28-coronavirus-updates-toronto-news)

Hundreds of millions of children worldwide have been denied the chance to learn and play at school. Anxiety and depression are soaring; on social media people proudly and publicly self-report that they have not gone outside for months. (https://www.washingtonpost.com/health/2020/05/04/mental-health-coronavirus/)

The lockdowns have punished all of us (except technology and social media companies, which are reporting record profits) enormously. Which might not matter if we had compelling evidence they worked.

Only we don't.

So the calls by some members of Team Apocalypse for *renewed* lockdowns – even *harder* lockdowns, in fact, as if we didn't do enough damage in the spring – might sound like a joke. Especially since hospitals even in the hardest-hit Sunbelt states are beginning to empty. But they're not a joke. They're serious – as the decision on Aug. 2 by the Australian province of Victoria to impose a new and draconian lockdown on Melbourne, a city with 5 million people, shows.

Lockdowns have failed as badly as the experts warned us they would, for precisely the reasons those experts spent their careers predicting. But the hysterics have learned nothing from the last four months.

Experience has shown that communities faced with epidemics or other adverse events respond best and with the least anxiety when the normal social functioning of the community is least disrupted.

Those words are as true now as they were in 2006. We have forgotten them once already this year.

We can't afford to make that mistake again.

Made in the USA
Las Vegas, NV
20 October 2020

10114236R00030